Miracle Sugars

The New Class of Missing Nutrients

RITA ELKINS, M.H.

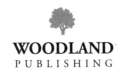

WOODLAND
PUBLISHING

For ordering or other information, please contact us:
Woodland Publishing
P.O. Box 160
Pleasant Grove, Utah
84062
Visit us at our web site: www.woodlandbooks.com
or call us toll-free: (800) 777-2665

The information in this book is for educational purposes only and is
not recommended as a means of diagnosing or treating an illness. All
matters concerning physical and mental health should be supervised
by a health practitioner knowledgeable in treating that particular condition. Neither the publisher nor the author directly or indirectly dis-
penses medical advice, nor do they prescribe any remedies or assume
any responsibility for those who choose to treat themselves.

ISBN 1-58054-354-5
Printed in the United States of America

Contents

Author's Note: Defending Against Bioterrorism

This booklet was written before the American tragedy of September 11, 2001. As a health reporter and author, I want to stress that while antibiotics save lives, they alone should not be relied on as the body's only defense against bacteria infections. Moreover, antibiotics should not be used for viral infections at all unless a secondary bacterial infection sets in.

The overuse of antibiotics now poses a threat as dangerous as the organisms they were designed to eradicate. Abusing antibiotic therapies has created a whole new class of super bugs that do not respond to antibiotic treatment. Granted, if one is exposed to very volatile bacteria, the body's innate defense mechanisms may not be able to overcome the infection. It is true, however, that fortifying the immune system prior to exposure certainly creates much better response and recovery odds. It would be detrimental to take antibiotics every day in order to cover that "just in case" encounter with an infectious bacteria. Doing so would actually harm our health. By contrast, taking certain nutritional supplements everyday can provide us with added protection and maximum immune mobilization without compromising our health.

Scores of natural products and supplements claim to boost and modulate the immune system and many of them do just that. It is my personal hope that medical practitioners and the general public alike will realize that we must approach infection before, rather than after the fact.

Glyconutritionals (biologically active sugars) are superb immune enhancers which can prepare and optimize our defense against serious infections of all kinds. They should be an integral part of anyone's immune fortification program. At the "Comprehensive Medical Care for Bioterrorism Exposure" congressional hearing on November 14th, 2001, in his opening statement, Dr. H. Reg McDaniel stated, "In instances of unusual, epidemic, or virulent infectious agent exposure, glyconutrient supplementation has been found effective for enhancing general immune functions and defense. When supplied at higher levels than available in nature, sugars needed for cellular synthesis can take innate defense systems to a much higher level that are effective against infectious agents."

Introduction to Glyconutrients

Virtually undetected until recently, the glyconutrients I call "miracle sugars" offer a new universe of health potential. Scores of studies have linked a deficiency of these extraordinary sugars to everything from lupus and diabetes to heart disease to cancer; from ADHD to infertility. Since they are so basic to the needs of every cell in the body, dozens of other illnesses have been linked to an imbalance of these sugars. This booklet attempts to explain how critical these sugars are for human health. As far as immune enhancement goes, they must be viewed as absolutely essential for maximum disease prevention and health maintenance.

All Sugars Are Not Created Equal

Question: If you were told that your diet was iron deficient and you were anemic, would you hesitate to take an iron supplement? Doubtful.

Question: If you were told that you lacked a group of necessary sugars to stay healthy and fight disease, would you hesitate to take them in supplement form? Maybe.

The difference is that you understand one and not the other. Originally, I had my own doubts about supplemental sugars. Since refined white sugar is considered by many to be public health enemy number one, my first reaction to using supplemental plant sugars to prevent and cure disease was "you've go to be kidding."

Fortunately, after studying the subject, I came to realize that we're not talking about table sugar at all. I discovered that there are over 200 carbohydrate monosaccharides in nature and they are **all** called sugars. Only a few of these, however, can be considered "necessary biologically active sugars."

Heralded as the vital missing link in our diets, researchers have identified up to eight specific and three metabolic intermediate biological sugars that most of us fail to obtain through our diets. In fact, the average American diet only supplies two of these sugars, creating what may be the most potentially serious nutrient deficiency we face.

In a very short time, I came to understand what ancient herbalists have known for generations—that plants rich in these special sugars have extraordinary immune-boosting powers. Along with our daily vitamin, mineral, and antioxidant array, we should be taking supplements containing these powerful saccharides. These sugars are absolutely essential for proper cellular survival and function. Without them, our cells, particularly our immune system cells, do not work at optimum levels.

Specific Carbohydrates Monosaccharides =
Biologically Active Sugars = Glyconutrients

Supplementing a variety of these sugars or "glyconutrients" on a daily basis helps correct the chemical imbalances that are causing a global epidemic—dysfunctional immunity—the cause of a myriad of devastating diseases. Moreover, it appears that correcting glyconutrient deficiencies may even help to reverse some genetic code malfunctions.

In the course of my own research over the last ten years, I have come to the conclusion that the cause of virtually every disease and disorder boils down to three things:

1. a malfunctioning immune system
2. free radical damage from bad fats, chemicals, UV rays, etc.
3. deficiencies of vital nutrients

Relatively unknown until recent years even to the scientific community, glyconutrients have the unique ability to address all three of these major modern-day health threats.

The marriage of these very specific sugar molecules with proteins and fats impacts virtually every cell's structure and function and may well be the greatest determinant of good health and longevity. It turns out that these sugars provide complex and sophisticated actions, giving cells the ability to transfer coded messages that sustain life and maintain health.

Back to the Future

Ironically, the future of our victory over disease may depend on looking back to the past. Even though the notion that biological sugar supplementation could prevent scores of diseases may raise some eyebrows, consider that much of what ancient medical practitioners prescribed has been validated by modern science.

For example, Greek and Roman physicians used liver extracts to treat poor eyesight. Today we know that liver is rich in vitamin A, which prevents the development of night blindness. The same correlation applies to vitamin C depletion and scurvy, low iron levels and anemia, as well as thiamine (vitamin B) deficiency and beri beri. Each of these conditions results from becoming deficient in one vital nutrient.

Once the importance of vital nutrients was recognized in disease prevention, food manufacturers began adding them to food. Vitamin D was added to milk to help prevent childhood rickets, a devastating disease that deformed the bones of countless children. Likewise, iodine has been routinely added to salt since 1930 to prevent goiter, an enlargement of the thyroid gland. Both of these diseases have virtually been eliminated.

The need for proper nutrition was sanctioned by the U.S. Congress with the passage of the Dietary Health and Education Act (DSHEA) in 1996. In the preamble they stated the following claims:

1) Improving the health status of U.S. citizens ranks at the top of the national priorities of the Federal Government.

2) The importance of nutrition and the benefits of dietary supplements to health promotion and disease prevention have been documented increasingly in scientific studies.

3) There is a link between the ingestion of certain nutrients or dietary supplements and the prevention of chronic diseases such as cancer, heart disease, and osteoporosis.

> Q: What is the most important nutrient for health maintenance?
> A: The one that's missing!

Could the reason that so many illnesses (especially immune and auto-immune-related) are on the rise is because we have become deficient in the special sugars discussed in this booklet?

The Golden Age of Glyconutrition

Simply stated, the Greek word *glyco* refers to "sweet." Hence, a glyconutrient is a biochemical that contains a sugar molecule. The prefix *glyco* can be placed in front of a fat, protein, or any molecule and suggests that a sugar is attached. Glycobiology is the study of the sugar portion of these proteins and fats.

Glycoprotein = Sugar attached to a protein
Glycolipid = Sugar attached to fat
Glycoform = Any sugar form

Like so many new frontiers in science, the role of these carbohydrates (sugars) was badly neglected and underestimated. They were at best considered a simple source of energy and at worst considered nothing more than a contaminant on the surface of the cell.

Virtually every cell in our bodies is covered with minuscule hair-like glycoforms. Until the invention of the electron microscope, scientists could not see these molecules on the surface of the cells. They could detect hairs (proteins and fats), but could not distinguish that on the surface of those hairs were trillions of other molecules—sugar molecules.

Glyconutrients are not vitamins, mineral, proteins, fats, herbs, enzymes or homeopathic drugs. They are carbohydrates. Just as there are essential proteins called amino acids and essential fats called fatty acids, glyconutritionals are the newly discovered class of necessary carbohydrate nutrients.

"The last decade has witnessed the rapid emergence of the concept of the sugar code of biological information. Indeed, monosaccharides represent an alphabet of biological information similar to amino acids and nucleic acids, but with unsurpassed coding capacity." (Acta Anatomica 4/1998)

Sugar-bound glycoforms work to keep our hormones in balance, to fight off disease invaders, to enable blood to clot, to give our cells their structural support network, and (perhaps most important of all) to create a complex cellular messaging system.

Today more that 20,000 research papers on glycoproteins a year, over fifty every single day, are published worldwide.

The "Healthy Sweets"

Sucrose is the "sweet" with which we are the most familiar, but it also happens to be the worst for our health. Sucrose is dangerously overused in America: the average American's annual consumption of refined white sugar (sucrose) has shot from 5 pounds in 1900 to 163 pounds today. Refined sugar is nothing but empty calories and does nothing for our health; however, there are other sugars that play a very important, beneficial role in our health. The "healthy sweets" we do need are as follows:

Glucose is readily available in our diets (converted from white sugar, fructose, and starchy foods) and in most cases is oversupplied in the form of sugar cane, rice, corn, potatoes, wheat, etc.

Galactose is readily available in our diets. It is obtained from the conversion of lactose (milk sugar) and is also easily obtained from dairy products **unless** you suffer from lactose intolerance.

Fucose is not readily available in our diets but is readily found in breast milk and in several medicinal mushrooms. It has numerous well-documented benefits for the immune system.

Mannose is not readily available in our diets. It plays a profound role in cellular interactions and has even been known to lower blood sugar levels. It is absolutely vital to proper immune defenses against microbial invaders and has a natural anti-inflammatory effect.

Xylose is not readily available in our diets. It is often seen in sugarless gums and candies. in that it has a sweet taste but does not cause tooth decay. It has recently been added to nasal sprays and appears to discourage the binding of allergens and pathogens to mucous membranes. It also has known antibacterial and fungal properties and may help prevent certain cancers.

N-acetyl-neuramic acid is not readily available in our diets but is another sugar that abounds in breast milk and dramatically impacts brain function and growth. It, too, boosts immune function and has documented antiviral actions. Interestingly, in certain disease states, the ability to digest this sugar is impaired.

N-acetyl-glucosamine is not readily available in our diets. It is particularly beneficial for cartilage regeneration and joint inflammation.

Glucosamine, a well-known natural medicine for arthritic conditions comes from this sugar compound. It has many more therapeutic effects and deficiencies or malfunctions of this sugar have been linked to diseases of the bowel.

N-acetyl-galactosamine is not readily available in our diets. It is the least known of the essential sugars although it appears to inhibit the growth of some tumors, and like the other sugars, plays an individual role in keeping cell communiqués clear and promptly delivered.

These sugars are so important to our health, that Mother Nature has made provisions to ensure we get them early on in life. Breast milk contains five of the essential sugars mentioned above. Emerging research continues to support how important breast-feeding is to human development—both short term and long term. The areas most noted as positively affected by breast milk nourishment are immune function and brain development.

> *FACT:* One reason that breast-fed babies are protected from infections is because breast milk is full of glyconutrients that may actually prevent infectious organisms from sticking to intestinal cells.

Sweet Messenger Molecules

Did you know that your health depends on the ability of cells to talk to each other? Virtually every bodily process that both protects and heals us involves certain intra- and inter-cellular transmissions. These coded messages control everything from wound healing to cancer cell destruction.

In the past it was thought that proteins supplied cells with these codes. Just a few years ago, however, scientists discovered that it was actually the sugar molecules found on their surface that formed the "words" cells use to communicate with their neighbors. When the body has the right supply and assortment of sugars to work with, it makes remarkable structures called "glycoforms." These glycoforms carry cellular codes and attach to the surface membranes of other cells of all kinds. When two cells of any type touch, the glycoforms on each cell actually speak to one another through their intricate sugar codes. If the body is lacking in these sugars, the code can be corrupted.

How Important is Cellular Communication?

What is the difference between these two words?

FAT   EAT

The difference is one tiny line at the bottom of the letter *E*. This tiny line, however, conveys an entirely different meaning. The same is true in cellular communication. When communication is good, things work the way they should. But what happens if written communication breaks down? What if you don't have all the letters you need to write a word? You send the wrong message. Similarly, if some sugars are missing, you can get sick.

Consider just one condition—rheumatoid arthritis. Certain cells of patients with arthritis have malformed glycoproteins that are missing only one sugar—galactose. The more of this sugar that's missing, the more severe the arthritis is. Arthritis is only one example. Malformed cell surface glycoforms are now known to be characteristic of many diseases.

> Saccharides are essential in virtually all intelligent interactions between the cells of the body; they're a critical part of the cell intelligence and activity. Glyconutrients affect how our cells form the structure of the body and the daily repair of our tissues. They play an important role in helping our body distinguish what belongs in it from what does not belong, and so they are vital to how our cells react to bacteria and viruses. Virtually every change within our multicellular bodies, from conception until death, is to some degree mediated by this language of sugars.
>
> *Dr. Emil I Mondoa, M.D.*, Sugars that Heal

Core Nutrition

Glyconutritionals could quite possibly be more important than any of the other nutrients. They lie at the core of your cell's ability to communicate all of their needs—even their need for other nutrients. A lack of any of these sugars can lead to body system malfunction and poor nutrient assimilation, simply because the need was not properly communicated.

Not only do the essential sugars work in cell-to-cell communication, they are also a vital part of the expression of the cell. The sugars that comprise this system break down the code and express it so it makes sense thereby prompting desired results. For this reason, scientists are moving past the Genome Project (identifying the genes) to Glynomics—how genes express themselves through sugars. It is possible that certain genetic defects are not defects at all. They may be due to genes that have not been able to express themselves properly.

Why You Should Take a Glyconutrient Supplement

- Do you get recurring colds and sore throats easily?
- Do you or other members of your family fight chronic infections?
- Does cancer run in your family?
- Would you like to make your family more disease-resistant with advanced immune support for life?
- Would you like to shorten the duration of infections without becoming dependent on antibiotics?

Modern Dietary Deficiencies

The human body requires water, vitamins, minerals, enzymes, proteins, fats, and carbohydrates to function properly. The foods we eat supply these macronutrients and come from a variety of sources. Once we moved away from the farm, however, and become a fast food society, the need for supplementation has now become mandatory.

Of the essential sugars, only two are readily available in our modern diets. In times past, we obtained a better array of glyconutrients. Actually many of the plants around the world that have a high glyconutrient content are known as "healing plants." Glyconutrients are found in the following ways:

aloe vera	certain mushrooms	echinacea
astragalus	yeasts	maize
saps	husks	pectins from fruits
gums	breast milk	some algae
garlic	coconut meat	certain herbs

> Knowledge of these sugars' functions could affect medicine far beyond improving drug doses and fighting cancer. Researchers are looking into how sugars influence the development of Parkinson's, Alzheimer's and infectious diseases like AIDS and herpes, to name a few. Sugars also seem poised to influence stem cell biology, organ transplantation and tissue engineering. If these promising areas of research prove successful, "sugars pills" will take on a whole new meaning.
>
> *Erika Jonietz*
> *from "Glynomics" in* Technology Review *10/2001*

There are several reasons why our modern diets and lifestyle actually provide us with less of the essential glyconutrients than our predecessors.

Green harvests, processed foods, preservatives, increased toxins, along with the limited variety of grocery store foods we eat, all reduce our supply of glyconutrients. Gradual soil depletion has also had an adverse effect on the quality of our fruits and vegetables. Of the necessary sugars, only glucose and galactose are abundantly supplied in our diets. Glyconutrient supplementation helps us get the extra glyconutrients we need.

Can the Human Body Make Glyconutrients?

Yes, we do have the ability to manufacture some glyconutrients, but to do so requires complex chemical pathways. The harmful effects of stress, toxins, poor nutrition, and genetic abnormalities in our metabolism can inhibit this conversion. Consequently, the number and structure of our glycoproteins may be impaired, which can lead to a number of serious health conditions common to our day.

Could these conditions be our modern-day scurvy or beri beri? Could the increase in disease states we see today actually be nothing more than nutritional deficiencies? Consider this—what if those deficiencies involved a class of nutrients that remained unknown until only ten years ago? If our assumptions are true, then it only stands to reason that these conditions could be dramatically treated with the missing nutrients.

Glyconutrients enhance tissue repair (wounds, sores, periodontal disease etc.), help to control the appetite, and work to curb chemical addictions. The inability to use these sugars properly has also been linked to cystic fibrosis and anemia.

The more we learn about virtually every disease or disorder, the more we realize that a malfunctioning immune system is the real and silent cause of everything from heart disease to obesity.

Glyconutrient Conversion

Glyconutrient sugars are absolutely vital for the body to function properly. In fact they are so important, that the body has a fail-safe mechanism that can convert them from one to another through a highly complex series of enzyme steps. Enzymes are like little conversion factories that reside within our cells. They change things inside the cell without changing themselves. Enzyme conversions require high levels of biochemical energy and can be interrupted by toxins, stress, drugs, processed foods, lack of proper enzymes, and age. When converting sugars, if any one of the fifteen different enzymatic processes necessary is interrupted, the whole cycle has to start all over again.

Even though the body can do that, having to do so on a regular basis creates stress, and the process can become more inefficient. It's like having to assemble a nut or bolt every time you needed one on an assembly line, as opposed to having them on hand as the cars rolled down the line. It is far more efficient for your body to obtain glyconutrients directly from your food or through supplementation, so they are immediately accessible for use. Glyconutrient supplementation can also free up the enzyme factories to do other vital conversions necessary for optimal cellular health.

Glyconutrients: The More, The Merrier

The more glyconutrients we can directly supply to the body, the more raw materials it has to work with to rebalance our immune networks, help drive our energy pathways, help sweep up dangerous oxidants, and control the sophisticated cellular reactions that determine whether we are healthy or sick. When given the right tools, the human body has an enormous capacity to correct and heal itself. Each cell needs all of the essential sugars. The fewer the body has to convert on its own, the faster its reaction time for promoting and maintaining health.

If we lack any one of the necessary biologically active sugars mentioned, glycoprotein structures can become weakened or altered. As a result, cellular messages may be full of errors. Glycoprotein molecules that lack critical sugars can transmit all kinds of faulty information, or worse yet, say nothing at all. Cancer cells could be allowed to grow unchecked because immune cells failed to recognize them.

When cells are given an adequate array of sugars to work with, the speed and efficiency of their continual contact with each other is greatly enhanced. When our glyconutrient levels are deficient, cells can become misguided, sluggish or even confused. When this happens, we become susceptible to disease. To make matters worse, our ability to heal is greatly compromised.

The Antioxidant-Boosting Action of Glyconutrients

By now, most of us know that the better we can "round up" harmful free radicals, the better off our overall health and longevity will be. These dangerous oxidant compounds can actually deteriorate body tissue and cause premature aging. Boosting the action of certain substances that clean our cells of these unstable molecules is a good thing indeed.

One of the best antioxidants is supplied by the body and is called glutathione. If we become low in glutathione, we can become vulnerable to degenerative diseases like diabetes and premature aging. Rola Barhoumi, Ph.D., and her research team recently reported that glyconutrient supplementation increased the level of gluthathione by 50 percent and prevented glutathione depletion in liver cells, where potentially harmful chemicals are detoxified.

> There are an increasing number of scientists who feel that the lack of these essential plant nutrients is related to the development of chronic disease of all kinds. There is increasing evidence that we need to take these nutrients as supplements for continued health and to help our bodies to regain health when we are deficient in these nutrients.
>
> *Walter W. Meyer, M.D.*

A Diet Deficiency Today is a Clinical Event Tomorrow

Today, six out of the top ten causes of death are diet related, and chronic degenerative diseases afflict over 120 million Americans. Cancer has moved from the tenth leading cause of death to number two, even after Richard Nixon's "War on Cancer" spent thirty billion dollars attempting to find a cure. Diabetes has increased 700 percent since 1959. Nearly fifteen million American adults suffer from asthma and the Environmental Health Commission predicts that number will increase to twenty-nine million by 2020. Twenty-one million Americans suffer from arthritis, and approximately fifty million Americans suffer from auto-immune diseases, with 75 percent of these being female. Many of these auto-immune conditions were practically nonexistent thirty years ago.

Look at the average diet of children today—soft drinks, processed cereal, pizza, candy, fast food and their favorite and often only source of vegetables: french fries. Could this be why are seeing a dramatic rise in ADHD, to the point where eight million American children need to be drugged daily? Autism has gone from 1 in 10,000 children to 1 in 150 in a just ten years. And adult-onset diabetes is occurring at epidemic rates in children as young as eight.

New Headlines in Medical Research

There can be no doubt that deficiencies of these vital nutrients can lead to serious problems. Scientists are continually discovering new links between viruses, bacteria, and the immune system and many of the most common and most dangerous diseases. Take a look, you might be surprised at what they're learning about the importance of a strong, balanced immune system.

ARE VIRUSES AND BACTERIA THE REAL CAUSE OF HEART AND KIDNEY DISEASE?

In the August 2000 issue of the *American Journal of Medicine*, scientists reported that the hepatitis C virus could show up as a kidney infection or as heart disease. Last year, Italian researchers reported that the reason cholesterol deposits stick to the walls of arteries might be due to an undetected infection that inflames blood vessel walls.

ARE BACTERIA TO BLAME FOR MS?

The July 1999 issue of *Annals of Neurology* reported that a common bacteria called *Chlamydia pneumoniae* was present in all the patients tested in the study with multiple sclerosis (MS). In addition, 30 percent of people with MS also harbor the herpes virus.

EPILEPSY LINKED TO ABNORMAL IMMUNE CELLS

In 1997, a group of scientists looked at a total of 135 people with epilepsy. More than 80 percent of these people had one or more abnormalities in their cellular immune defenses.

ALZHEIMER'S DISEASE LINKED TO IMMUNE SYSTEM DYSFUNCTION

An article in a 1994 issue of *Progress in Drug Research* reported that Alzheimer's disease may be linked to an abnormal antibody response to a portion of nerve cells in the brain.

A HIDDEN VIRUS THAT CAUSES OBESITY

Researchers at the Department of Nutrition and Food Science at Wayne State University in Detroit reported in August of 2001 that increased fat stores have been linked to the presence of a virus.

IS ARTHRITIS REALLY A JOINT INFECTION?

Dutch scientists recently reported that chronic arthritis might have a bacterial connection. In fact, if you suffer from rheumatoid arthritis, which is considered an auto-immune disease, your disease may have been triggered by a prior infection that may have over stimulated immune responses which, in this situation, needed to be suppressed.

IS MALE INFERTILITY DUE TO *E. COLI* BACTERIA STICKING TO SPERM?

A German study in the July 1993 issue of *Fertility and Sterility* reported that *E. coli* can actually adhere to sperm causing them to clump together.

Immune System Assault and Battery

Modern living is making it harder and harder to maintain a healthy immune system. Here are just some of the forces working against it.

Poor nutrition. "Empty calories" is a term that aptly describes the typical American diet. Even a mild deficiency of iron and selenium can cause suppressed immunity, and Americans are typically low in both.

High-fat diets. In a 1993 report published in *Progressive Food and Nutrition,* scientists found that excessive fat intake impairs immunity.

Pollution. A recent report published in *Environmental Pollution and Neuroimmunology* stated that the combined influence of various factors (chemical agents, radiation, stress) may lead to immunodeficiency in the form of respiratory and inflammatory disease. Hundreds of studies show that toxic chemicals impair immune defenses.

Stress. Stress releases biochemicals that suppress immune function putting us at higher risk for bacterial, viral and fungal infections. Our emotional landscape impacts immunity. One study reported in a 1997 issue of *Psychosomatic Medicine* stated that posttraumatic stress suffered after Hurricane Andrew had dramatically reduced killer cells in test subjects.

Prolonged stress weakens or impairs immune response, making us vulnerable to infections, auto-immune diseases and even cancer. In a recent study published in a 2000 issue of *Psychological Medicine,* researchers reported that episodes of serious stress experienced early in life may predispose a woman to breast cancer.

Antibiotic resistance and "super bugs". Once considered miracle drugs, antibiotics are now abused to the point they pose a major health threat worldwide. Bacteria are now outwitting potent antibiotics creating the risk of global infections that won't respond to the best of the high-tech drugs. In a June 12, 2000 press release. The World Health Organization announced that almost all major infectious diseases are slowly becoming resistant to existing medicines.

> **FACT:** A study on the effects of glyconutritionals on candida showed that using only one glyconutrient had almost no affect; a partial blend had a kill rate of almost 50 percent, but using a complete blend of saccharides containing the known sugars required for glycoprotein and glycolipid synthesis in cells, had a kill rate of 95 percent.

Low natural killer cell levels. NK (natural killer cells) provide our first line of defense against invaders. A low NK cell count means a much higher risk of disease and tissue degeneration. Today we are able to measure the number of natural killer cells, and the news is not good.

In addition, the constant barrage of free radicals, alcohol, tobacco, dieting, international travel, eating disorders, prescription drug side effects, day care, food additives, aging, lack of sleep, poor digestion and elimination continually weakens our natural immune defenses.

Diseases Associated With Impaired Immunity

OVERACTIVE IMMUNE DISORDERS

asthma

eczema

food allergies

urticaria (hives)

rhinitis

pollen and grass allergies

AUTO-IMMUNE DISEASES

lupus

psoriasis

scleroderma

rheumatoid arthritis

multiple sclerosis

type 1 diabetes

INFLAMMATORY DISORDERS

fibromyalgia

celiac disease

ulcerative colitis

Crohn's disease

irritable bowel syndrome

UNDERACTIVE IMMUNE DISORDERS

viral and bacterial infections

hepatitis B and C

shingles

tuberculosis

colds and flu

HIV

herpes simplex 1 and 2

sinusitis

chronic fatigue syndrome

OTHER

stress-related disorders

cancer

type 2 diabetes

benign prostatic hyperplasia

Glyconutrients and the Immune System

Remember that all disease states begin at the cellular level. Our bodies are simply an accumulation of cells that must work together in harmony. Each has it's own structure, function, and duty to perform.

Healthy Cells = Healthy Tissues = Healthy Organs = Health Bodies

In other words, if our cells (the basic building blocks of life) do not receive the right mix of nutrients, they do not stay healthy. This leads to a cascade effect, which ultimately ends in some diseased condition. Let's examine this from the viewpoint of a glyconutrient deficiency.

> As our diet only provides two of the eight essential sugars necessary to make the required glycoproteins, the body must synthesize the other six from internal resources. If deficiencies in any of these sugars occur, the needed glycoproteins are not synthesized, limiting the cell membranes ability to carry out the necessary cell-to-cell communications. This break in communication inhibits the cell's natural ability to defend against disease and illness.
>
> *Tony Serio, M.Ed.*

The Consequences of Cell Miscommunication

We know that a glyconutritional deficiency can lead to a breakdown in our cells' ability to properly communicate their needs. Consequently, our immune cells may fail to recognize, warn and mount an attack on invaders, which leads to higher risk of infection. Also, cell miscommunication can lead to faulty signals, causing the immune system to mistake healthy tissue as a foreign invader called an antigen; i.e., auto-immune diseases, pollen allergies, etc. But perhaps the most pernicious result of cell miscommunication results in the failure of the immune system to recognize replicating mutated cells, which if unchecked, inevitably leads to cancer.

The Consequences of Glyconutrition

Complete glyconutrition provides immune balance, fortification, and maintenance. We don't want an overactive immune system . . .we don't want an underactive immune system . . . what we want, is an immune system that is "just right."

If your immune system is too weak, you become susceptible to bacterial, viral, fungal and parasitic infections. If your immune system is over activated, you become susceptible to auto-immune diseases, where immune armies attack human tissue, mistaking it for the enemy; i.e. lupus, type 1 diabetes, rheumatoid arthritis, psoriasis, Crohn's disease, etc.

Imagine an immune system that is watchful and strong enough to immediately respond to threatening infections. Herbal practitioners have known for millennia that botanicals rich in these special sugars can spike immune chain reactions to better combat infections and boost healing. Glyconutritionals are very unique because they are immune system modulators. This means glyconutrient supplementation can help to correct an overactive immune system (auto-immune diseases), boost an under active immune system (chronic or recurring infections), and keep immune armies in tip-top shape for exceptional disease prevention.

How Do They Do That?—The Antigen Factor

All cells including infectious microorganisms carry "ID Tags" called antigens on their surface. Each of these individual molecular signatures tells our immune generals whether the intruder is friend or foe. If foe, the antigens stimulate the immune system to produce antibodies to act against it. Amazingly, immune defense cells recognize and respond to thousands of antigens. These "ID Tags" are written in glycoforms on the surface of the cells and use the sugar code to pass the information.

> **FACT:** Scientists are discovering that diseases once thought to be unrelated to infectious invaders are really caused by microorganisms that either fail to trigger the proper immune response or over stimulate that response.

Immune cells roam throughout the body touching other cells and ask three questions:

1. Are you me (part of this body) and are you OK?
2. Are you me and are you not OK (do you need help)?
3. Are you not me and need to be eliminated or destroyed?

These questions and their answers are translated through the sugar code found on each cell surface. Depending on the response obtained, immune cells:

1. Leave the cell alone
2. Send for help to repair or protect the cell
3. Call in the troops to kill of the foreign invader or cancer cell

Correct immune response is complicated by the fact that many infectious agents routinely mutate, confusing the immune system. This explains why we can catch multiple colds and flu over the course of time. Each time there is a mutation, a new antigen needs to be developed. This requires a complex communication cycle between T and B immune cells. The faster this occurs, the faster the immune system can prevent and heal damage from mutated infectious agents. Once the new antibody signature is learned by the immune system, it stays in memory forever. Having a ready supply of glyconutrients may help the body speed up this process.

Scientific Research Backing Glyconutrition

At this writing, the glycosciences are considered cutting edge research. There are over 20,000 studies conducted annually on glycoforms alone. Researchers from universities and major pharmaceutical companies realize the importance of this new discovery. Breaking the "sugar code" will mean a tremendous advancement in health and medicine.

Studies confirm that the eight essential biologically active sugars can accomplish amazing results. The following are just a few examples of the exciting possibilities of glyconutrition:

1. Dramatically raises natural killer cell and macrophage count against infectious organisms
2. Activates immune T-cell activity only when invaders or antigens are present
3. Decreases cell death in chronic fatigue syndrome
4. Dramatically elevates disease resistance in weakened individuals
5. Acts as antioxidant compounds, which boost the collection of dangerous free radicals
6. Protects the body against toxin and pollutant exposure
7. Slows premature aging
8. Decreases inflammation in diseases like rheumatoid arthritis
9. Helps immune cells recognize invaders due to a mutual "sugar exchange" of info
10. Enables cellular components to stick to each other initiating the right reactions

Adaptogenic Glyconutrients vs. Pharmaceuticals

Most doctors will agree that the body (when functioning properly) has an extraordinary ability to heal itself. In fact, our immune systems are continuously destroying viruses, bacteria, fungi and even cancer cells to keep us disease-free. Likewise, when we fail to supply that system with vital nutrients, it fails to protect us, not only from diseases, but from premature aging as well.

Ancient medical practitioners knew what we have to relearn today— that some plant compounds have a brain. In other words, glyconutrient supplements and other adaptogenic plant compounds can enter the body and act according to need and individual situation. They either stimulate reactions to heal when you are sick, or work in other pathways to prevent illness. Simply stated, they help the body **adapt** to its particular health challenge and environment. To put it another way—they initiate healing rather than just masking symptoms. No prescription high-tech drug can do that.

Today hundreds of millions of dollars are being spent by at least fifteen pharmaceutical companies researching the potential of carbohydrate drugs, vaccines and delivery systems. Recent television commercials are even referring to future drugs that will be delivered directly to the diseased cells, leaving the healthy cells alone. Synthesizing the sugar communication code and coating the drug, so it would then seek out only the diseased cells could accomplish this goal which would be an exceptional medical breakthrough. An article in the January 1993 edition of *Scientific American* states, "The day may not be far off when anti-adhesive drugs, possibly in the form of pills that are both sugar coded and sugar loaded will be used to prevent and treat infections, inflammation, the consequences of heart attacks and perhaps even cancer."

Remember, drugs don't cure disease. Even with drugs—the body does the healing. Drugs are designed to offer symptom relief by blocking or intercepting natural biological activity until the body fixes itself. The medical profession will openly admit they have no cure for any auto-immune disease, but only treat to offer relief to its victims.

Drug symptom relief, however, can be costly. All drugs are toxic and can have serious side affects. In fact, more than 100,000 deaths related to the use of legally prescribed medications occur every year in the U.S. This is now the fourth leading cause of death, and although it goes relatively unnoticed, consider that this is comparable to a 270-passenger jet crashing everyday for a year and killing everyone on board. Taking drugs should never be a casual decision. Taking multiple drugs can be deadly. If you are taking drugs, please inform your doctor of all the drugs you are using before adding more.

Fortunately, many people are also turning to non-drug alternatives, exercise, improved diets and nutritional supplements. *JAMA* reports that 50 percent of Americans have gone to alternative care physicians. Fifty to seventy percent of Americans are taking nutritional supplements. Make no mistake, drugs and antibiotics can be life saving tools in our medical arsenal when used properly, but they should not be used for health maintenance and disease prevention.

Immune Vigilance—Top Priority

Glyconutritional supplementation may represent the best of preventive medicine. In today's health-threatening environments we need to act before, not after the fact. Keeping our glycoprotein profile in tip-top shape is one of the smartest ways to keep our immune systems vigilant.

Supplying the body with the glyconutrient essential sugars may help resolve, and more importantly, prevent:

viral infection	fungal infection	parasitic disease
auto-immune disease	malignant disease	bacterial disease
microbacterial disease	neurological disease	

Faulty Cell Communication and Disease

There is no question that when cellular communications break down, so does our health. When immune cells mistake the good guys for the bad guys and engage in cell-to-cell combat, auto-immune diseases can develop.

> Glycobiology has achieved critical breakthroughs in the medical field, primarily by addressing what could be the greatest plague in health care today—auto-immune diseases. Multiple sclerosis, arthritis, diabetes, Crohn's disease and colitis are just a few of these diseases.
>
> *Neecie Moore, Ph.D.*

EXAMPLES OF FAULTY DATA TRANSMISSIONS.

M.S. Immune cells are mis-instructed to attack the myelin sheathes that cover our nerves.

lupus. Immune cells are mis-instructed to attack organs like the liver or the skin.

psoriasis. Certain skin cells don't get the "quittin time" message and continue to grow into thick plaques.

type 1 diabetes. Immune cells are mis-instructed to attack islet cells in the pancreas that make insulin.

rheumatoid arthritis. Immune cells are mis-instructed to attack cartilage cushions in joints.

Crohn's disease. Immune cells are mis-instructed to attack bowel tissue.

As you can see from this varied list, immune attack cells can get faulty messages and end up destroying tissue located anywhere in the body.

How do we prevent such a terrible misuse of the immune system? Research tells us that monosaccharide supplementation could actually prevent auto-immune diseases. Several studies by Dr. T. Feizi and his associates suggest that a dietary deficiency of certain sugars may spark the development of auto-immune diseases. In fact, the Newkirk study published in a 1996 issue of *Clinical and Experimental Immunology* (among others) found that galactose deficiencies were common in almost all cases of auto-immune disease.

> **FACT:** Glyconutrient supplementation can increase NK cell activity as much as 50 percent in healthy people and up to 400 percent in people with compromised immune systems.

Remember that cellular messages direct the show. In other words, if the "glycogram" telegraphs the wrong message, immune attack cells will turn on the body. Glycomolecules actually tell immune cells when and where to mount an attack.

Human tissue that is continually attacked by mis-informed immune cells is subject to chronic inflammation that causes pain and cell destruction, this can lead to prolonged illness or even death. For example, immune cells in diseases like lupus may choose to attack liver tissue eventually making the organ non-functional.

Overactive Immune Disorders

There are thousands of papers demonstrating glyconutritional immune system support. Below are some conditions associated with a malfunctioning immune system.

ASTHMA AND ALLERGIES: MISGUIDED INFLAMMATION

Inflammation is nature's way of protecting us from infection. For example, when that pesky sliver gets under your skin, macrophages and other white blood cells rush to the site to fight the alien invader. As a result, the area becomes red, swollen and tender until the rescue operation is complete.

Sometimes the inflammatory response command is issued when it shouldn't be. Asthma and most allergies deal with exaggerated inflammatory responses. In asthma, irritation causes the bronchial tubes in the lungs to constrict and eventually breakdown.

Allergies occur when immune cells mistakes a substance like pollen for a foreign invader. In this case, the inflammatory process causes histamine to be released from mast cells (causing congestion, itching, sneezing, etc.). Typically, antihistamine drugs are used to inhibit this response. Interestingly, one of the essential eight does the same thing.

> **FACT:** Providing the immune system with the right glyconutrients helps it recognize infectious organisms more readily. Remember, it is the "glyco" or sugar portion of both our immune cells and invading organisms that transfer messages.

Researchers belonging to the Faculty of Pharmaceutical Sciences, Kumamoto University, Japan, discovered that the sugar called N-acetyl-neuraminic acid blocked the release of histamine (the culprit chemical in allergic reactions).

Concerning these studies, the Lefkowitz research team of the University of South Florida says, "Taken in their entirety, the above studies suggest that glyconutrients, because of their saccharide composition, may represent a new approach to inhibiting the inflammatory response.

This is an area we believe definitely merits further research. Inhibiting inflammation would benefit numerous diseases including asthma." The possibilities for glyconutrient supplementation as a therapy for allergic and asthmatic inflammation are truly exciting.

Auto-Immune Disorders

RHEUMATOID AND OSTEOARTHRITIS

In rheumatoid arthritis, the process of inflammation goes into overdrive and our own immune cells destroy cartilage, which normally cushions and lubricates our joints. While osteoarthritis is considered a result of "wear and tear," rheumatoid arthritis is considered an auto-immune disease. Although hidden viruses and bacteria have been suspected as the real cause of rheumatoid arthritis, the jury is still out.

A recent study found that L-fucose is low in people with rheumatoid arthritis and described it as a promising treatment since it is "a safe and simple natural sugar."

Interestingly, the lowest levels of fucose have been linked to the most advanced cases of rheumatoid arthritis. According to the work of Doris Lefkowitz, Ph.D., the severity of rheumatoid arthritis has also been linked to low galactose levels and vice-versa. According to her report, the vicious cycle of inflammation seen in arthritis is caused by abnormal "cross-talk" between immune cells. Mannose is also crucial for joint protection

Two other essential sugars (N-acetylglucosamine and N-acetylgalactosamine) also work to sweep up destructive free radicals in joints that form during any inflammation. These sugars also keep well-intentioned but misguided immune attack cells from sticking to healthy cells.

N-acetylglucosamine: A famous joint-friendly sugar. If you suffer from osteoarthritis, which is not considered an auto-immune disease, and take NSAID's (non-steroidal anti-inflammatory drugs) for pain and swelling, the natural anti-inflammatory effect of glyconutrients can also be of great benefit. Glucosamine has already gained celebrity status for its ability to stimulate the regeneration of cartilage in damaged joints and has been the subject of countless studies. It does indeed prompt healing, reduce swelling and increase flexibility.

LUPUS

Lupus, another auto-immune disease, has also been linked to abnormalities and deficiencies of mannose-binding proteins. The same thing was found in people with dermatomyosisits.

FACT: In 1996, the Sullivan study published in *Arthritis and Rheumatism* concluded that a low level of mannose-binding proteins may make a person susceptible to lupus. This conclusion stresses the vital role that mannose plays in staying healthy.

As is the case with all auto-immune diseases, the production of "auto-antibodies" causes the immune system to invade healthy tissue. Because glyconutritionals are so profoundly involved in "getting immune cell messages straight," supplementation should be considered.

DERMATOMYOSITIS

Dermatomyositis (a disease of connective tissue with arthritis-like symptoms) is characterized by sugars whose structures changed after a parasitic infection. We've already established that whenever the "glyco" or sugar part of a molecule is altered, communication channels can break down and the wrong commands can be given. This is one of several auto-immune diseases that show the same profile—a lack of dietary sugars—the inability to absorb them—or abnormalities in their structures.

When deciding how to tackle an auto-immune disease, consider this statment by Neecie Moore, Ph.D.: "Following on evidence, it seems likely that a balanced intake of the various monosaccharides may provide an effective preventive measure for auto-immune diseases. But the best news is that supplementing the diet with glyconutrients can provide great benefits without forcing patients into long-term use of any of the steroidal medications with their many adverse side effects."

> **FACT:** Scientists at the Glycobiology Institute at Oxford recently discovered macrophages (the immune cells that eat invaders) have mannose receptors that activate immune attacks.

MULTIPLE SCLEROSIS

MS has been linked to the inability to absorb xylose or the presence of abnormal galactose molecules. Interestingly, the myelin sheath that covers our nerves and is attacked by immune cells in MS contain galactose. This being the case, galactose and xylose supplementation may have a corrective effect.

One study of a group of people with MS found that supplements containing fats and galactose improved symptoms.

DIABETES (TYPE 1 AND 2)

Sugars to fight a blood sugar disease? As we all know, the incidence of both type 1 and type 2 diabetes is skyrocketing and health practitioners are very concerned (a 500 percent increase over the last twenty years). Glucose is seen as the enemy in diabetes. Ironically, the therapeutic use of other sugars may actually benefit diabetics.

For example, in type 1 diabetes, glyconutrients other than glucose may actually stimulate the pancreas to produce more insulin. Moreover, it does so without causing the damaging side effects of high blood glucose levels (retinal destruction). Scientists at the Metabolic Research Laboratory in

Glyconutrition in Action

I am eighty-five years old and have practiced medicine for over fifty years. When I first heard of glyconutritionals I refused to even consider them because of the broad range of benefits I was being told that they delivered. I kept my mind closed for a over a year until one day I got to thinking—"What could possibly help that many conditions in the body?" and it hit me—"The Immune System." If glyconutritionals really were 'missing nutrients' then replacing them would help the immune system communicate and work better and that would do it. I started taking a glyconutrient product. When I started, I wrote a list of everything that was wrong with me. I listed twenty things. I wasn't being neurotic—just scientific. After four months, twenty of the twenty-one had dramatic improvements—but I still wasn't convinced. I became convinced when a muscular dystrophy patient of mine also had a dramatic turn around using glyconutritionals. I have taken care of this patient for fifty years. She has been in total care since she was two years old and she's fifty-three now. She was in total atrophy and was on oxygen twenty-four hours a day. Now, for the first time in her life she is feeding herself, brushing her teeth, and she even paints. She is off her oxygen several hours a day and hasn't had an infection of any kind even though her roommate and nurses taking care of her have all had the flu. Miracle sugars—now I'm convinced.

Dr. Rayburn Goen

Minneapolis have found that mannose and galactose (among other glyconutrients) have proven their ability to increase insulin secretion.

In a study published in the November 1997 issue of *Proceedings of the Fisher Institute for Medical Research* reported people with type 1 diabetes who were given dietary compounds including glyconutrients (mannose and others) reported a dramatic improvement in their health, not to mention a decrease in vision problems, better wound healing, less infections, and lower blood pressure. In addition, some of the participants were able to lower their insulin medications.

RECENT RESEARCH NEWS

- Glucose injections have also been tested and show promise for ovarian cancer.
- Arabinogalactan, which has a galactose backbone, can stimulate the immune system enough to block the spread of cancer cells.
- Injections of fucose in laboratory test animals has shown promise for breast cancer.
- When scientists added sugars including D-mannose, D-ribose, and D-glucosamine into the drinking water of mice carrying with tumor cells, their survival rate was increased and tumor rate decreased.
- Xylose supplements may prevent cancer of the digestive system.

Preventing blindness caused by diabetes. One of the worst complications of diabetes is the destruction of the retina by high levels of circulating blood sugar. The delicate retinal screen is literally "eaten away" by damaging proteins created by the presence of high blood glucose.

In a study published in 1995, researchers at the Ophthalmology Department of Harvard University suggested that mannose might be able to substitute for glucose. Mannose has the ability to become the energy source for cells without the risk of eyesight damage. Of equal importance is that it could also work to stimulate the pancreas to produce more insulin, thereby lowering the amount of insulin needed to control this disease.

Underactive Immune Disorders

CANCER

One in every three Americans will develop cancer. Doctors diagnose 1.2 million cancer cases every year in this country, and that number is going up, not down. Of these, six in ten people will die within five years.

WHAT IS CANCER?

Cancer is the uncontrolled growth of abnormal cells permitted to reproduce due to serious immune collapse. Cancer is permitted to grow unchecked because our immune surveillance system falls asleep.

Immune guard cells normally identify and destroy cancer cells. Immune cells called B-lymphocytes produce antibodies designed to destroy malignant cells. In some people, the system breaks down, so cancer cells do not trigger normal alarm mechanisms.

People with faulty immune responses are at a much higher risk of developing cancer. Because we can't avoid exposure to pollution, pesti-

> For cancer to start and continue growing, it must out-maneuver the many long arms of your immune defenses. The immune system is both your first and last defense against cancer.
>
> *John Bailar, M.D., Ph.D., former Editor-in-Chief of the* Journal of the National Cancer Institute

cides, additives, ultra-violet rays, etc., it is crucial that we boost our natural immune defenses to protect us against cancer.

Why plant-rich diets fight cancer. We all know that our diets are intimately linked to the formation of cancer, and yet most of us continue to eat poorly. One reason that a diet rich in fresh fruits and vegetables is cancer-preventive is due to its rich glyconutrient and phytochemical content.

The current popularity of high-protein, high-fat, low-carb or no-carb diets puts our immune systems at even more risk for phytonutrient depletion.

Glycoproteins and cancer: The latest word. Could the real cause of cancer boil down to the abnormal formation of glycoproteins due to glyconutrient depletion? Research tells us that when levels of the essential eight sugars become low, cancer can result. Some scientists have concluded that the abnormal structures of glycoproteins could be a tell-tale sign of cancer formation.

Abnormal mannose and N-acetylglucosamine sugars have been found in breast and colon cancer cells. In addition, a lack of monosaccharide sugars have been linked to the spread of cancer cells throughout the body. Dr. Hirayama, who has extensively studied these sugars, suggests that cancer of the gastrointestinal tract may result from a lack of monosaccharide intake.

FACT: In study results published in a 1985 issue of Cancer Research, scientists reported that the formation of cancer cells in the stomach and colon is unmistakably related to deformed or absent sugar molecules. Scientists at the University of South Florida have found that the rate in which these cancers spread may be linked to glyconutrient availability.

The cancer glyconutrients. Glyconutrients that have proven anti-tumor properties include mannose, glucose, galactose, glucosamine and fucose.

Mannose: Manager of macrophages. Proteins that carry mannose sugars on their surface can actually stimulate macrophages to literally "devour" cancer cells. Moreover, when mannose binds to these cells, it activates macrophage action, and also initiates the secretion of other substances (like interferon), which alert and reinforce other immune defenses. By so doing, the growth of cancerous tumors is inhibited.

The cancer track record. Glucose injections have also been tested and show promise for ovarian cancer. Arabinogalactan, which has a galactose backbone, can stimulate the immune system enough to block the spread of liver cancer cells. Injections of fucose in laboratory test animals have shown promise for breast cancer.

When scientists added sugars including D-mannose, D-ribose, and D-glucosamine into the drinking water of mice with tumor cells, their survival rate was increased and tumor rate decreased. Xylose supplementation may prevent cancers of the digestive system.

Dr. Ronald Klatz in his book *Advances in Anti-Aging Medicine, Vol. 1* (1996) reported that a study known as "Norman's Rats" found that 40 percent of rats that had no defense against cancer and were given injections of just one of the essential eight sugars showed "tumor regression and complete recovery."

Four ways glyconutrients fight cancer. First, they stimulate macrophage and immune killer cells to destroy cancer (first line of defense). Second, they increase the production of substances like interferon to target and destroy malignant cells.

> **FACT:** Scientists at the Department of Cellular and Molecular scientists in London confirmed that abnormal cellular sugar structures can cause antibodies to attack healthy tissue.

Third, they activate T-cells to recognize invaders and destroy them (second line of defense). Fourth, they help to regulate when cells die off (apoptosis). When this safety mechanism fails, cancer cells are allowed to keep replicating.

It is also believed that glyconutritional supplementation may enhance the effects of chemotherapy for cancer patients.

Can glyconutrient supplementation prevent cancer? More than one study shows that galactose and glucose may prevent liver cancer. According to a study published in the March 1997 issue of *Anticancer Research*, supplementing the body with galactose decreases the number of liver tumors.

INFECTIONS

Our cells aren't the only ones with sugar components on their surface. Infectious organisms do, too. So when they enter the body, all kinds of chattering between friend and foe cells occurs and the fight begins. The Lefkowitz research team has extensively studied glyconutrients and they put it this way: "Through the interactions of these surface carbohydrates, which act as cell-to-cell communication signals, microorganisms can gain access to our body, start to multiply, and cause disease."

Various sugars such as mannose can supply the raw materials that actually interrupt the process of infection. They accomplish this by first, slowing down the reproduction of disease organisms; and second, boosting immune cell activity (especially macrophages).

VIRAL DISEASES

Even with all of our sophisticated drugs, viruses have managed to evade destruction. More than 400 viruses are known to infect human cells. Like bacteria and fungi, they too have glycoproteins that reside on their surfaces. For example, the influenza virus has sugar compounds on its surface that help it pierce through a healthy human cell.

BACTERIAL INFECTIONS

Bacteria (normally treated with antibiotics) have sugar-bound proteins called adhesins that stick to the sugar portion of our cells and vice versa. This "sticking" is considered the first step in the process of a bacterial invasion. The Lefkowitz research team points out that bacteria with the ability to engage in this exchange include *E. coli*, *N. gonorrhea*, *Mycobacterium tuberculosis*, and some strains of salmonella and staphylococci. Keep in mind that a defect in the molecules could impede this "sticky sugar" interaction. Plant sugars fight bacteria in two vital ways. First, they keep bacteria from reproducing and colonizing; and second, they potentiate immune cell defense capabilities

BRONCHITIS

Scientists actually administered the sugar N-acetylneuramine through an inhaler to laboratory test animals with bronchitis and concluded that it helped to minimize the infection.

TREATING AND PREVENTING INFLUENZA

Scientists at the Biomolecular Research Institute in Victoria Australia reported in April 10th, 2001 issue of *Protein Science* that N-acetylneuraminic acid was an anti-flu virus agent. Another study suggests that it may be a very effective flu treatment if given early enough. Like bacteria, flu viruses continually mutate so each year, our immune systems have to deal with a whole new viral ball game. One animal study published in a 1995 issue of *Antimicrobial Agents and Chemotherapy* reported that a N-acetylneuraminic acid mixture was up to 1,000 times more effective in fighting the influenza virus than potent anti-viral drugs.

CHRONIC FATIGUE SYNDROME (CFS)

This debilitating syndrome has baffled doctors and continues to evade a cure. Some experts believe that the Epstein-Barr virus causes it, while others classify it as an auto-immune disorder.

The addition of supplemental glyconutrients stimulated glycoprotein performance, increased natural killer cell levels, stopped premature cell death, and gave the immune system what might be called an "overhaul." Interestingly, the symptoms of chronic fatigue and fibromyalgia are strikingly similar, including fatigue, poor sleep patterns, aches and pains, weakened immunity, and depression.

EAR INFECTIONS

According the World Health Organization, antibiotic-resistant bacteria are due, in part, to the over-prescription and misuse of antibiotics for one of the most troublesome childhood illnesses—ear infections. To make matters worse, ear infections are increasing and the use of new and more powerful drugs are failing to control their recurrence.

Studies strongly suggest that using mannose can help inhibit the progress of an ear infection. In fact one study published in the November issue of *Molecular and Cellular Biochemistry* reported that using mannose in combination with antibiotics was better than antibiotic treatment alone.

According to another report found in the December 2000 issue of *Vaccine*, using xylitol dramatically reduced the number of ear infections in children by inhibiting the growth and attachment of *Streptococcus pneumoniae* in the tubes that run from the throat to the ear.

> **FACT:** Immune cells called neutrophils that cause inflammation are present in asthma attacks. Researchers at the Hahnemann University School of Medicine confirmed that neutrophils are suppressed by mannose or N-acetylglucosamine. Once again, it all boils down to normalizing misdirected immune reactions.

HIV, AIDS, AND ANTIBODY ATTACK

Glycoproteins are critically important in the study of AIDS. Recent studies confirm that sugars may play a major role in how the AIDS virus spreads. Japanese researchers at the AIDS research center in Tokyo have found that mannose, fucose and N-acetylglucosamine actually inhibited the HIV virus. In addition, according to a study in a 1990 issue of the *American Journal of Clinical Nutrition*, a xylose deficiency was found in AIDS patients suggesting that xylose supplementation may boost better energy levels.

In a study published in a 2000 issue of *Phytotherapy Research* and conducted at the Department of Microbiology at the University of Texas at Antonio, researchers reported that aloe vera polymannose showed significant activity against the coxsackie virus by dramatically boosting antibody attack. In fact, they concluded that aloe polymannose can "immunopotentiate" antibody production against not only these viruses but herpes as well.

LIFE-THREATENING STREP INFECTIONS

Dr. Michael Schlacter, an internist specializing in pulmonary diseases at Mountain View Hospital in Las Vegas, credits immediate and massive glyconutrient supplementation for saving the life of Greg Letourneau.

Greg was admitted and diagnosed with streptococcal toxic-shock syndrome and was given little chance of survival. In the face of complete organ failure and with the family's approval, Dr. Schlacter administered very concentrated doses of a glyconutrient mixture rich in mannose and other sugars through Greg's feeding tube. Within hours, he was out of danger. Greg, his family, and Dr. Schlacter believe that intensive glyconutrient therapy saved his life.

URINARY TRACT INFECTIONS

This infection sends scores of women to their doctors and is typically treated with potent antibiotic drugs. Most cases are caused by the contamination of the urinary tract by *E. coli* bacteria. Keep in mind that *E. coli* bacteria have sugar molecules that enable them to stick to the cells that occupy the lining of the bladder.

Dr. E. Michaels and his researcher team concluded that a combination of mannose and glucose sugars was able to reduce the severity of a urinary tract infection with twenty-four hours.

YEAST (CANDIDA)

While more research is needed on the workings of sugars and fungi, we do know that yeast *(Candida albicans)* infections interact with our body cells through the action of mannose-containing proteins found on their surface. Scientists announced in the April 22nd issue of the *International Journal of Immunopharmacology* that mannose does indeed speed up the destruction of yeast organisms.

Macrophages bind to the mannose molecules found on candida. In one study conducted at the Department of Botany and Microbiology at the University of Kuwait, the addition of mannose and N-acetylglucosamine was so significant that it protected laboratory test mice against the reproduction of yeast in the digestive tract. Our ability to fight other fungal infections, such as athlete's foot, nail fungus, etc., may also be enhanced through glyconutrient immune stimulation.

Inflammatory Disorders

FIBROMYALGIA

Like chronic fatigue syndrome, fibromyalgia continues to puzzle medical practitioners. Characterized by chronic muscle and tissue tenderness typically affecting certain trigger points, treating fibromyalgia with drugs has seen limited success. Impaired muscle cell repair and regeneration has been linked to fibromyalgia.

Low serotonin levels may play a role in this disease. Glyconutrients greatly impact the way brain chemicals are produced and used. In fact, tests have found that when essential sugars are taken away from certain brain chemicals, their uptake by surrounding cells is decreased.

Fibromyalgia may also be linked to a hidden virus—a fact that may signal weakened immune function. If so, the essential eight sugars, which have demonstrated impressive anti-viral action, would again be an appropriate therapy.

In a study published in the January-March issue of *Integrative Physiological and Behavioral Science*, a group of test subjects with fibromyalgia and chronic fatigue syndrome who consumed a nutritional supplement containing freeze-dried aloe vera extract (rich in acetylated mannans), glyconutrients and other natural compounds reported significant improvement in their symptoms.

ULCERATIVE COLITIS

Studies showed that people with colitis have problems with the monosaccharide (sugar) function in their colons. Even more telling is that over half of the healthy subjects in one study published in *Clinical Science* contained all eight essential sugars in the mucus lining of the bowel as compared to barely a fourth of the people with bowel disease.

ULCERS

One study showed that test animals were protected from stress-related stomach ulcers by glycoproteins, which exerted a protective effect on the stomach lining. They stated that "this protective force breaks down during restraint stress, as indicated by reduced gastric adherent mucus and a low level of carbohydrate components in the gastric secretion.

Sugar molecules make up the mucous lining of the stomach that protects it from acids, bacteria, chemicals, etc. Dr. J. F. Forstner's research has found that peptic ulcer formation is connected to defective links between sugar molecules. Moreover, we know now that *H. pylori* bacteria cause protective stomach mucus to break down, and an ulcer can result. This also suggests that glycoprotein malfunction caused the immune system to fail.

Other Conditions and Diseases

LEARNING DISORDERS AND BRAIN CELL CARBOHYDRATES

Brain cells are extremely dependent on well-functioning glycoproteins to operate at maximum efficiency. For this reason, making sure that the essential sugars "or brain building blocks" are continually supplied only makes good sense.

In a study of an eight-year-old boy with dyslexia published in the August 1997 supplemental issue of the *Journal of the American Nutraceutical Industry*, using a combination of glyconutrients combined with other phyto (plant) chemicals resulted in an advance from low to middle level school performance. It was also noted that the child was less agitated and frustrated.

ALZHEIMER'S DISEASE AND OTHER BRAIN DISORDERS

The brain's sole source of fuel comes from glucose. If blood glucose levels dip, so does our ability to think. Interestingly, in a 1994 issue of *Gerontology*, scientists reported that brain cells of test subjects with Alzheimer's disease had a serious problem metabolizing glucose. In another report published in 1993 in the *Journal of Internal Medicine*, consistently low levels of blood glucose were also associated with Alzheimer's disease.

Fucose, galactose and N-acetylneuraminic acid supplementation have all been associated with better memory recall. In fact, in animal studies conducted at La Trobe University in Australia fucose was actually able to overcome artificially induced amnesia.

ADD AND ADHD

Parents that live with ADHD (Attention-Deficit Hyperactive Disorder) are only too familiar with the link between white sugar and behavior. Children with ADHD often react with extreme behavior after eating sweets, suggesting that their ability to properly metabolize sugar may be impaired. In addition, miscommunication between glycoproteins may be at the heart of the problem. If an ADHD child fails to digest sucrose (white sugar) properly, it's possible that child may lack the right enzymes needed to produce all eight essential sugars from glucose.

In a study published in the January-March 1998 issue of *Integrative and Physiological and Behavioral Science*, researchers tested seventeen children who had been diagnosed with ADHD. For three weeks, a glyconutrional supplement that included all of the essential eight sugars was given. After that time period, another plant-derived supplement was added. The authors of the study concluded, "Most importantly, the dietary supplements we used significantly reduced the number and severity of ADHD symptoms of children, whether they were taking or not taking methylphenidate (Ritalin)."

In another study published in the November issue of *Proceedings of the Fisher Institute for Medical Research*, researchers concluded, "This study replicates the earlier findings of Dykman et al., showing that glyconutrional products improve the health of ADHD subjects and reduce the number and severity of symptoms."

FAILURE TO THRIVE AND GENERAL WASTING SYNDROMES

Considered one of the most tragic of childhood diseases, FTT cause the body to literally waste away. Seen in adults in cases of AIDS or cancer and called *cachexia*, both disorders have been linked with the inability of the body to use dietary nutrients.

Research data cited by Tom Gardiner Ph.D. indicates that, "a recent study in FTT children demonstrated that supplementation of their diets with glyconutritional substances, including some that act as immune system modulators, resulted in definite improvement of their FTT symptoms." He points out that one of the more direct causes of FTT symptoms are due to the failure of glycoproteins to transport sugar, something that can actually start in the placenta.

The inability of the body to metabolize these sugars (genetic enzyme deficiencies) inevitably leads to impaired immune function. mannose, galactose, fucose and N-acetylnereuraminic acid are all involved, and Gardiner concludes that because these sugar molecules play such a crucial role in functions surrounding FTT, their supplementation may be critical in preventing the malfunctions that cause this terrible disease.

GASTROINTESTINAL DISORDERS

The gamut of gastro-glitches that plague great numbers of Americans runs from simple indigestion, heartburn and constipation, to irritable bowel syndrome, gastric ulcers and stomach and colon cancer.

German studies confirm that changes in sugar molecules found in the mucus membranes of the large intestine have a very important link to the development of inflammatory bowel diseases. Plant lectins found in mannose, galactose and fucose play a key role in protecting us from the poisonous chemicals that are generated in the colon.

INFERTILITY

Infertility rates in both men and women are rising. The rather startling possibility that the inability to conceive may be due to *E. coli* bacteria that stick to sperm making them clump together was supported by a German study published in the July 1993 issue of *Fertility and Sterility*. What they concluded—this phenomenon is controlled and can be prevented by D-mannose. We also know that the ability of sperm to penetrate an egg relies on a series of enzymatic reactions that depend on the presence of certain cell sugars and proteins.

In addition, researchers at the Department of Obstetrics and Gynecology at North Shore University Hospital in New York found that mannose increases the efficiency of sperm. They concluded that exposing human sperm to mannose ligands and D-mannose offers a new way to study male infertility.

HEART DISEASE: AN INFLAMMATORY CONDITION?

Heart disease is now the leading cause of death and 63 percent of the women and 50 percent men will die from their first attack.

There is a growing body of evidence that suggests that instead of cutting out and reaming our "pipes" to deal with cholesterol deposits, we should be adding certain nutrients to the liquid that flows through them. New studies show that bacteria associated with other diseases is also causing inflammation on artery walls making them much more likely to collect cholesterol.

In the February 1999 issue of *Science*, chlamydia (a bacteria) and herpes (a virus) have been linked to heart attacks. Most of us are routinely exposed to these microorganisms, which in some cases, decide to attack the lining of our arteries.

These studies imply that the inability of the immune system to eradicate these invaders may lie at the real "heart" of heart disease. The question is **why** does this happen in some people? Could sugar molecules that lack their protein "spouse" be to blame?

Sugarless proteins may prompt the development of heart disease. Scientists have discovered that groups of people who were heart attack survivors had a much higher count of proteins that were minus attached sugars. These "headless" proteins were often missing their glucosamine sugar mates. Interestingly, researchers at the National Institute of Food and Nutrition in Warsaw discovered that their "sugarless" state correlated to higher cholesterol and blood fat levels.

What does this all mean? It tells us that keeping heart muscle continually supplied with glyconutrients is vital to its protection and repair. It even suggests that a lack or malfunction of these sugars and proteins may initiate the beginnings of heart disease—the collection of cholesterol on artery walls.

PARASITIC DISEASES

The amoebal parasite called acanthamoeba can cause serious eye infections and like *E. coli*, sticks to mannose receptors on healthy cells. We know that mannose and N-acetyl-d-glucosamine can inhibit amoeba-induced infections.

Enhancing Athletic Endurance with Glyconutrition

An article in the May 1999 issue of *Muscle & Fitness Magazine* entitled "What Can Glyconutrients Do For You" reported that by boosting maximum immune responses, glyconutrients help to avoid the immune breakdown often seen after intense training.

Tom Gardiner Ph.D. reports that physiochemical stress such as increased temperature, lowered pH, increased calcium ion concentration, and decreased oxygen content are particularly prominent during exercise. Strenuous or prolonged physical exercise can weaken immune response.

In addition, dangerous free radicals are formed at a more rapid rate when we exercise. It is thought that by avoiding the severity of these internal breakdowns, gains in lean body mass may be enhanced or better maintained. It is also thought that glyconutrient supplementation may increase the efficiency of an athletic workout so less exercise might render the same effect as more.

Your Daily Diet and Glyconutrients

THE BEST NATURAL SOURCES OF THE PRIMARY GLYCONUTRIENTS

It is no coincidence that many of the sources of glyconutrients have been used all around the world for centuries as healing medicinal compounds.

BREAST MILK

Mother Nature, M.D. certainly knows what she's doing. Breast milk contains five of the essential sugars—fucose, galactose, N-acetylneraminic acid, N-acetylglucosamine and Glucose—a fact that in and of itself supports the notion that the human body requires many different kinds of sugars to develop properly. Breast milk is a veritable immune potion, and although we understood the importance of antibody transfer between mother and child, we do not yet appreciate the profound health implications of its sugar array.

A study published in a 1998 issue of *Biological Neonate* reported that several different glycoproteins found in breast milk can protect breast-fed babies against infection by microorganisms. The report explained that these compounds actually bind to bacteria like *E. coli* and to rotavirusus. In addition, they revealed that these sugar compounds actually inhibit the binding of the HIV virus to a host cell. Their conclusion—these sugars provide protection against several disease-causing organisms and the toxins they produce.

ALOE VERA

Known as the "Potted Physician," aloe contains mannose, galactose and arabinose. The leaves of this plant are extremely rich in polysaccharides (long chain sugars) that give aloe its healing and anti-infection properties when used both externally and internally. Its mannose content is what also makes aloe a superior immune booster.

Aloe's beneficial properties. Studies show that aloe has antifungal, antiviral, antibacterial, anti-allergy, and anti-inflammatory properties. Aloe inhibits arthritis inflammation and partially inhibits HIV virus replication. Aloe vera is also synergistic with AZT and Acyclovir. Aloe blocks histamine production, controls symptoms of asthma, kills candida, heals peptic ulcers, reduces *E. coli* in mice, blocks salmonella adhesion in chickens, protects liver from chemical injury, has significant anti-tumor activity, and can help prevent the replication of viruses in the body.

ARABINOGALACTAN

Sap is sugar. Many of the sources of the glyconutritionals come from the saps and gums of trees and plants. Arabinoglactan can be obtained from the *Larix decidua* or larch tree and can also be found in a variety of vegetables and fruits such as tomatoes, corn, carrots, coconut as well as in the immune-stimulating herb we know as echinacea. Echinacea also contains galactose and arabinose.

Arabinogalactan's beneficial properties. Studies show that arabinogalactan has anti-inflammatory and anti-allergy properties. It also stimulates NK cells, blocks liver lectins (proteins that are binding sites for monosaccharides) that mediate tumor metastisis, blocks settling of sarcoma L01 tumor cells, and protects intestinal mucosa against disease and cancer promoting agents. Arabinogalactan also aids in the recovery of chronic fatigue, increases beneficial intestinal bacteria, decreases otitis media ear infections, and decreases levels of viral DNA similar to human hepatitis B. It also aids in the recovery of hepatitis B & C and in the recovery of MS. And finally it also stimulates NK cell cytotoxicity (the ability to kill cells).

Just this year, a study published in *Plant Molecular Biology* reported that arabinogalactan proteins (AGPs) play an important role in cell-cell recognition, and programmed cell death (what keeps cells from growing into malignant tumors). Another recent study confirmed that the these sugars positively impact the chemical nature of fecal matter, which can dramatically impact colon health and the kind of bowel bacteria that is present. In addition, arabinogalactins have proven anti-viral actions against hepatitis B.

ASTRAGALUS GUMMIFER

The stems and branches of astragalus shrubs are rich in galactose, arabinose, xylose, fucose, rhamnose, and galcturonic acid, and proteins.

Studies show that it is an antioxidant, diuretic, anti-inflammatory, and a hypotensive. Astragalus inhibits tumor growth, offsets the immune suppression of cancer chemotherapy. It stops colon bifidus fermentation, decreases intestinal transit time, stimulates synthesis of antibodies, delays the natural aging process of blastocysts (fertilized egg cells) by one third, increases number of stem cells in the marrow and lymph, and stimulates stem cell development into active immune cells. Long-term astragalus use heightens activity of spleen cells and reduces the duration of common cold from 4.6 days to 2.6 days.

GUM ACACIA

Extracted from the African acacia tree, gum acacia contains arabinose, galactose, rhamnose and glucuronic acid. Studies show that it lowers triglyceride production, lowers serum cholesterol. controls colon bifidus fermentation, improves beneficial intestinal flora, promotes healing of irritated respiratory tract tissue, and promotes healing of irritated gastrointestinal mucosa.

GUM GHATTI

Obtained from the sap of the indian sumac. It contains galactose, arabinose, mannose, xylose, and glucuronic acid benefits. Studies show that it lowers cholesterol and is excellent for bifidus fermentation.

LIMU MOUI

A marine vegetable native to Tonga, limu moui contains the glyconutrients galactose, mannose, and xylose. It has been shown to enhance immunity, fight allergies, inhibit blood clotting, decrease cholesterol levels, improve and support liver function, and to detoxify the body.

MEDICINAL MUSHROOMS AND BETA GLUCANS

Edible mushrooms have been used medicinally in China from ancient times to present. They contain an immune-enhancing sugar compounds known as lentinant (a polysaccharide that contains beta-glucans), which stimulates the body's white blood cells to, not only devour invaders, but to detoxify or "clean up" the toxins they leave behind. They are rich in glucose, galactose and mannose. They are known to boost immune chemicals such as interleukin-1 and 2 and helper-T and NK natural killer cells to fortify and expand the immune system's ability to respond to invaders (infectious, carcinogenic, etc). They also suppress inappropriate immune reactions, have anti-tumor properties and the unique ability to act as "immunomodulators." Beta-glucans also prevent the decline of white blood cell in people undergoing chemotherapy and radiation.

Numerous studies have report that beta-glucans fight cancer and tumor growth, can extend cancer survival time, fight infection in people who have suffered traumatic injuries, improve recovery from radiation treatments, boost wound healing and protect people with severe infections from going into shock. Beta-1,3 glucans stimulate immune action without making the system overactive (a plus for people with autoimmune diseases). Beta-glucans also enable immune defenses to better fight bacteria, viruses, fungi, parasites and toxic substances.

PECTINS

Used to give jellies and jams their firmness, pectin comes from fruits like apples, pumpkins and tomatoes. Pectins are a form of fiber and have proven cholesterol-lowering properties. They are also considered a source of glyconutrion. The fact that most of us fail to eat enough fruit once again supports the notion that we fail to obtain glyconutrients from our diets. In addition, one of the reasons that a diet high in fruit is considered cancer-protective is due, in part, to the glyconutrient content of fruit pectin.

A report in the *Journal of Physiological Biochemistry* confirmed that the pectin in oranges and apples significantly decreased cholesterol levels in the liver. A 1997 report found in a well-known cancer journal revealed that apple pectin has definite anti-cancer effects in the colon.

Glyconutrient Product Availability

Several glyconutrient products can be purchased at health food stores or through product distributors. Some supplements specialize in a particular glyconutrient such as the glucosamine products for joint relief. Ideally, taking a daily supplement that provides the best and most complete array of the glyconutrients is recommended. Remember, the more of these vital missing nutrients you can add back to your diet, the fewer your body will have to manufacture for optimal cellular communication.

Glyconutrients are available in freeze-dried products, extracts, loose powder or capsulated forms. Look for high-quality supplements that not only contain a varied array of sugars but offer them at adequate levels. Products that are guaranteed and offer standardized and stabilized active ingredients are preferable. In addition, look on the label for a telephone number, so you can contact the manufacturer directly if you have any questions or concerns.

Glyconutrient Safety Issues

As a rule, if you have any health condition or are taking any medication, you should consult your doctor before taking any supplement. Supplementation with glyconutrients is considered generally safe and nontoxic. These sugars are considered foods. However, anyone with a blood sugar disorder should consult their physician. If you are allergic to yeasts or fungi, you may need to avoid some products. If you experience fast or irregular breathing, skin rashes, hives, or itching after taking any supplement, call your doctor or the company's customer service department. You should also consult your doctor before taking any supplement if you have kidney or liver disease or are pregnant or nursing. At this writing, the safety of these supplements in pregnancy or in infants who are breast fed has not been established.

References

Adam, E et al. "Pseudomonas aeruginosa II lectin stopshuman cillary beating:therapeutic implications of fucose" American Journal of Respiratory Conditions, Care and Medicine (1997):155(6):2102-2104.

Ahmad, I et al. "Design of liposomes to improve delivery of amphotericin-B in the treatment of aspergillosis" Mole Cellular Biochem (1989 Nov 23-Dec 19):;91(1-2):85-90.

Benoff, S et al. "Induction of the human sperm acrosome reaction with mannose-containing neoglycoprotein ligands" Molecular Human Reproduction (1997 Oct):3(10).

Benton, D. "Case Report: Observed Improvement in Develpmental Dyslexia Accompanied by Supplementation with Glyconutritionals and Phytonutritionals" JANA, Journal of the American Nutraceutical Association (August, 1997): suppl 1, 13-14.

Berger, V et al. "Dietary specific sugars for serum protein enzymatic glycosylation in man" Metabolism (1998 Dec):47(12):1499-503.

Bhavanandan, V "Cancer-associated mucins and mucin-type glycoproteins" Glycobiology (1991 Nov):1(5):493-503.

Bond, A et al. "Distinct oligosaccharide content of rheumatoid arthritis-derived immune complexes" Arthritis and Rheumatism (1995 Jun):38(6):744-9.

Bouhnlk, Y et al "Administration of transgalacto-oligosaccharides increases fecal bifidobacteria and modifies colonic fermentation metabolism in healthy humans" Nutrition (1997):127(3):444-448.

Brandelli, A et al. "Participation of glycosylated residues in the human sperm acrosome reaction: possible role of N-acetylglucosaminidase" Biochem Biophys Acta (1994 Feb 17):1220(3):299-304.

Braaten J et al "Oat beta-glucan reduces blood cholesterol concentration in hypercholesterolemic subjects" European Journal of Clinical Nutrition Jul1994:48(7):465-74.

Brennan, F et al. "TNF alpha—a pivotal role in rheumatoid arthritis?" British Journal of Rheumatolgy (1992):31:293-298.

Brinck, U et al " Detection of Inflammtion and neoplasia associated alterations in human large intestine using plant/invertebrate lectins, glaectin-1 and neoglycoproteins" Acta Anatomica (1998):161: 219-233.

Burmester G et al. "Mononuclear phagocytes and rheumatoid synovitis. Mastermind or workhorse in arthritis?" Arthritis and Rheumatism (1997):40:5-18.

Chandra, R "Nutrition and the immune system: an introduction" American Journal of Clincal Nutrition (1997): 66:460-63S.

Chihara G "Recent progress in immunopharmacology and therapeutic effects of polysaccharides" Developmental Biological Standards 1992;77:191-7.

Cimoch, P et al. "The in vitro immunomodulatory effects of glyconutrients on peripheral blood mononuclear cells of patients with chronic fatigue syndrome" Integrative Physiological and Behavioral Science (1998 Jul-Sep):33(3):280-7.

Clamp, J et al. "Study of the carbohydrate content of mucus glycoproteins from normal and diseased colons" Clinical Science (Colch) (1981 Aug):61(2):229-34.

Crowe, S et al "2-deoxygalactose interferes with an intermediate processing stage of memory", Behavioral and Neural Biology (1994 May):61(3):206-13.

Dabelsteen, E "Cell surface carbohydrates as prognostic markers in human carcinomas" Journal of Pathology (1996 Aug):179(4):358-69.

Davidson M et al "The hypocholesterolemic effects of beta-glucan in oatmeal and oat bran: A dose-controlled study" Journal of the American Medical Association Apr1991:265(14): 1833-9.

de Felippe Junior et al "Infection prevention in patients with severe multiple trauma with the immunomodulator beta 1-3 polyglucose (glucan)" Surgical Gynecology and Obstetrics Oct1993:177(4): 383-8.

Dekaris, D et al. "Multiple changes of immunologic parameters in prisoners of war. Assessments after release from a camp in Manjaca, Bosnia" JAMA Journal of the

American Medical Association (1993 Aug 4):270(5):595-9.

Dhurandhar, N "Increased adiposity in animals due to a human virus" Interantional Journal of Obesity and Related Metabolic Disorders (2000 Aug): 24(8):989-96.

Djeraba, A et al. "In vivo macrophage activation in chickens with Acemannan, a complex carbohydrate extracted from Aloe vera" International Journal of Immunopharmacology (2000 May):22(5):365-72.

di Luzio N et al "Comparative evaluation of the tumor inhibitory and antibacterial activity of solubilized and particulate glucan" Recent Results of Cancer Research 1980:75:165-172. "Drug resistance threatens to reverse medical progress" Press Release, WHO World Health Organization/41 (12 June 2000).

Dwek, R et al. "Glycobiology: the function of sugar in the IgG molecule" Journal of Anatomy (1995):187:279-292.

Dykman, Kathryn and Dykman, Roscoe "Effect of Nutritional Supplements on Attention-Deficit Hyperactivity Disorder Integrative Physiological and Behavioral Science" (Jan-March, 1998): 33(1): 49-60.

Dykman, Kathryn and McKinley, Ray "Effects of Glyconutritionals on the Severity of Attention- Deficit Hyperactivity Disorder" Proceedings of the Fisher Institute for Medical Research (November, 1997): 24-25.

Dykman, K et al. "The effects of nutritional supplements on the symptoms of fibromyalgia and chronic fatigue syndrome" Integrative, Physiological and Behavioral Sci (1998 Jan-Mar):33(1):61-71.

Ercan, N et al. "Effects of glucose, galactose, and lactose ingestion on the plasma glucose and insulin response in persons with non-insulin-dependent diabetes mellitus" Metabolism (1993 Dec):42(12):1560-7.

Famularo, G "Infections, atherosclerosis, and coronary heart disease" Annals of the Italian Medical Institute (2000 Apr-Jun):15(2):144-55.

Feizi, T. and Larkin, M "AIDS and glycosylation" Glycobio (Sept 1990): 1(1): 17-23.

Feizi, T. "Significance of Carbohydrate Components of Cell Surfaces, Auto-immunity and Auto-immune diesease" CIBA Foundation, Symposium Series. (United Kingdom: Wiley-Interscience Publications, 1987), 43-57.

Flogel, Lvi et al. "Fucosylation and galactosylation of IgG heavy chains differ between acute and remission phases of juvenile chronic arthritis" Clinical and Chemical Laboratory Medicine (1998):36:99-102.

Forstner, J. "Intestinal mucins in health and disease" Digestion (1978):17(3):234-63.

Fukuda, M "Cell surface carbohydrates: cell-type specific expression. Molecular Glycobiology (Oxford: IRL Press, 1994).

Gardiner, T "Dietary xylose: absorption, distribution, metabolism, excretion (ADME) and biological activity" GlycoScience & Nutrition (2000): 1 (S):1-2.

Gardiner, T "Dietary fucose: absorption, distribution, metabolism, excretion (ADME) and (2000): 1(6): 1-4.

Gardiner, T "Dietary galactose: absorption, distribution, metabolism, excretion (ADME) and (2000): 1(7): 1-4.

Gardiner, T "Dietary N-acetylgalactosamine (GalNAc): absorption, distribution, metabolism, excretion (ADME) and biological activity". GlycoSci & Nutr (2000): 1(8): 1-3.

Gardiner T. Dietary N-acetylneuraminic acid (NANA): absorption, distribution, metabolism, excretion (ADME) and biological activity. GlycoScience & Nutrition 2000; 1(10): 1-3.

Gardiner T. Dietary mannose: absorption, distribution, muetabolism, excretion (ADME) of eight known dietary monosaccharides required for glycoprotein synthesis and cellular recognition processes.

Gardiner, T "Absorption, distribution, metabolism, and excretion (ADME) of eight known dietary monosaccharides required for glycoprotein synthesis and cellular recognition processes: summary" GlycoScience & Nutrition (2000):1(12):1-7.

Gardiner, T "Biological activity of eight known dietary monosaccharides required for glycoprotein synthesis and cellular recognition processes: summary" GlycoScience & Nutrition (2000):1(13):1-4.

Gardiner, T. "Dietary glucose: absorption, distribution, metabolism, excretion (ADME) and biological activity" GlycoScience & Nutrition (2000):1(18):1-4.

Gardiner, T. "Glyconutritional implications in fibromyalgia and chronic fatigue syndrome" Glycoscience and Nutrition, (June 3, 2000) 1(21).

Gardiner, T "Gyconutritionals Implications in Failure-to-Thrive Syndrome" Glycoscience and Nutrition,, (2001): 2:1.

Gaspar Y et al "The complex structures of arabinogalactan-proteins and the journey towards understanding function" Plant Molecular Biology 2001 Sep:47(1-2):161-76.

Gauntt, C et al. "Aloe polymannose enhances anti-coxsackievirus antibody titres in mice".Phytotherapy Research (2000 Jun):14(4):261-6.

Gauntt, C et al. "Glyconutritionals: Implications for Recovery from Viral Infections" Glycoscience and Nutrition (2001): 2:2.

Ghannoum, M et al. "Protection against Candida albicans gastrointestinal colonization and dissemination by saccharides in experimental animals" Microbios (1991):67(271):95-105.

Gibson, J et al. "Sugar nucleotide concentrations in red blood cells of patients on protein- and lactose-limited diets: effect of galactose supplementation" American Journal of. Clinical Nutrition (1996):63:704-708.

Glaser, R and Kiecolt-Glaser, J "Stress-associated immune modulation: relevance to viral infections and chronic fatigue syndrome" American Journal of Medicine 1998):105(3A):355-425.

Gordon, Garry MD "Heart Disease, America's No. 1 Killer" Explore (1999) 9(4-5).

Grevenstein, J. et al. "Cartilage changes in rats induced by Papain and the influence of treatment with N-acetylglucosamine" Acta P Belgica (1991): 57:2 157-61.

Gupta, J et al "Multiple sclerosis and malabsorption"American Journal of Gastroenterology (1977 Dec):68(6):560-5.

Hakomori, S "Aberrant glycosylation in cancer cell membranes as focused on glycolipids: overview and perspectives" Cancer Research, (1985): 45: 2405-2414.

Hakomori S. "Tumor malignancy defined by aberrant glycosylation and sphingo(glyco)lipid metabolism" Cancer Research (1996 Dec 1):56(23):5309-18.

Hitchen, P et al. "Orientation of sugars bound to the principal C-type carbohydrate-recognition domain of the macrophage mannose receptor" Biochemistry Journal (1998 Aug 1):333(3):601-8 .

"The influence of industrial environmental pollution on the immune system. New ideas of immunorehabilitation " International Conference on Environmental Pollution & Neuroimmunology (1995): 9.

Ironson, G et al "Posttraumatic stress symptoms, intrusive thoughts, loss, and immune function after Hurricane Andrew" Psychosomatic Medicine (1997 Mar-Apr):59(2):128-41.

Jacobs, J and Bovasso, G "Early and chronic stress and their relation to breast cancer" Psychological Medicine (2000 May):30(3):669-78.

Jorgensen, F et al. "Ivlodulation of sialyl Lewis X dependent binding to E-selectin by gly-coforms of alpha-i-acid glycoprotein expressed in rheumatoid arthritis" Biomed.Chron (1998):12:343-349.

Josephson L et al "Antiviral activity of a conjugate of adenine-9-beta-D-arabinofura-noside 5'-monophosphate and a 9 kDa fragment of arabinogalactan" Antiviral Therapy 1996 Aug:1(3):147-56.

Kahlon, J et al. "Inhibition of AIDS virus replication by acemannan in vitro" Molecular Biotherapy (1991 Sep):3(3):127-35.

Kai, H et al."Anti-allergic effect of N-acetylneuraminic acid in guinea-pigs" Journal of Pharmaceuticals and Pharmacology (1990 Nov):42(11):773-7.

Kamel, Lvi and Serafi, T "Fucose concentrations in sera from patients with rheumatoid arthritis" Clinical Experimental Rheumatology. (1995): 13:243-246.

Kamel, M et al. "Inhibition of elastase enzyme release from human polymorphonuclear leukocytes by N-acetyl-galactosamine and N-acetyl-glucosamine" Clinical Experimental Rheumatology (1999) 1 9 (9):17-21.

Kelley, D and Daudu, P "Fat intake and immune response" Progressive Food and Nutritional Science (1993)17:41–63.

Klatz, Ronald Adv in Anti-Aging Med, Vol. 1 (Ronald M. Klatz, Editor, 1996), 181-203.

Kobata, Akira "Function and pathology of the sugar chains of human immunoglobulin G. Glycobiology (September 1990), I(1): 5-8.

Kossi, J et al. "Effects of hexose sugars: glucose, fructose, galactose and mannose on wound healing in the rat" Eur Surg Res (1999):31(1):74-82.

Kotler, D et al. "Preservation of short-term energy balance in clinically stable patients with AIDS" American Journal of Clinical Nutrition (1990 Jan):51(1):7-13.

Landin, K et al. "Low blood pressure and blood glucose levels in Alzheimer's disease. Evidence for a hypometabolic disorder" Journal of Internal Medicine (1993 Apr):233(4):357-63.

Lefkowitz, D et al. "Effects of a glyconutrient on macrophage functions" International Journal of Immunopharmacology (2000 Apr):22(4):299-308.

Lefkowitz, Doris "Glyconutritionals: implications for rheumatoid arthritis" Glycoscience and Nutrition (April 15, 2000) 1(16).

Lefkowitz, Doris "Glyconutritionals: Implications in Asthma" Glycoscience and Nutrition, (2000): 1:15.

Lefkowitz, Stanley S. and Lefkowitz,, Doris L. "Glyconutritionals: implications in antimicrobial activity" Glycoscience and Nutrition (2000): 1:22.

Lefkowitz D et al. "Neutrophilic myeloperoxidase-macrophage interactions perpetuate chronic inflammation associated with experimental arthritis" Clinical Inonmomol (1999):91:145-155.

Lhermitte, M et al. "Structures of neutral oligosaccharides isolated from the respiratory mucins of a non-secretor (0, Le a+b-) patient suffering from chronic bronchitis" Glycobiology (June 1991) 1(3): 277-293.

Maihotra, R et al. "Glycosylation changes of IgG associated with rheumatoid arthritis can activate complement via the mannose-binding protein" Nat. Med. (1995):1:237-243.

Mansell P et al al "Macrophage-mediated destruction of human malignant cells in vivo" Journal of the National Cancer Institute Mar1975:54(3):571-80.

Matsuda, K et al. "Inhibitory effects of sialic acid- or N-acetylglucosamine-specific lectins on histamine release induced by compound 48/80, bradykinin and a polyethylenimine in rat peritoneal mast cells" Japanese Journal of Pharmacology (1994 Jan):64(1):1-8.

Mawle, A et al. "Immune responses associated with chronic fatigue syndrome: a case-control study" Journal of Infectious Diseases (1997):175(1):136-141.

McAnalley, B and Vennum, F "The potential significance of dietary sugars in management of osteoarthritis and rheumatoid arthritis: a review" Proceedings of the Fisher Institute of Medical Research (1997):1:6-10.

McDaniel, Candace, et al. "Effects of Nutraceutical Dietary Intervention in Diabetes Mellitus: A Retrospective Study" Proceedings of the Fisher Institute for Medical Research (November, 1997): 19-23.

Meyer, Walther W. M.D. E-mail: wwm-nutrimed@tds.net

Michaels, E et al. "Effect of D-mannose and D-glucose on Escherichia coli bacteriuria in rats" Urol Res (1983):11(2):97-102.

Mondoa, Emil MD. Sugars That Heal. (Ballantine Books, 2001).

Morikawa K et al et al "Induction of tumoricidal activity of polymorphonuclear leukocytes by a linear beta-1, 3-D-glucan and other immunomodulators in murine cells" Cancer Res. Apr1985:45(4):1496-501.

Moulton, P "Inflammatory joint disease: the role of cytokines, cyclooxygenases and reactive oxygen species" British Journal of Biomedical Science (1996):S3:317-324.

Mullin, B et al. "Myelin basic protein interacts with the myelin-specific ganglioside GM4 Brain Res (1981 Oct 5):222(1):218-21.

Murray, Robert K. Harper's Biochemistry. 24th ed. (Lange, 1996), 648-67.

Olszewski, A et al. "Plasma glucosamine and galactosamine in ischemic heart disease" Atherosclerosis (1990 May):82(1-2):75-83.

Petersen, M et al ."Early manifestations of the carbohydrate-deficient glycoprotein syndrome" Journal of Pediatrics (1993 Jan):122(1):66-70.

Peterson J et al "Glycoproteins of the human milk fat globule in the protection of the breast-fed infant against infections" Biological Neonate 1998:74(2):143-62.

Petruczenko A "Glucan effect on the survival of mice after radiation exposure" Acta Physiol Pol. May1984:35(3):231-6.

Prone Mice" Clinical and Experimental Immunology (Nov. 1996):106: 259-64.

Pugh, N et al. "Characterization of Aloeride, a new high-molecular-weight polysaccharide from Aloe vera with potent immunostimulatory activity" Journal of Agriculture and Food Chemistry (2001 Feb):49(2):1030-4.

Rest, R et al. "Mannose inhibits the human neutrophil oxidative burst" Jour Leukic Biol (1988):43:158-164.

Ringsdorf, W et al"Sucrose, neutrophilic phagocytosis and resistance to disease" Dental Survey (1976):52(12):46.

Robinson R "Effects of dietary arabinogalactan on gastrointestinal and blood parameters in healthy human subjects" Journal of the American College of Nutrition 2001 Aug:20(4):279-85

Ryan, D et al. "GG167 (4-guanidino-2,4-dideoxy-2,3-dehydro-N-acetylneuraminic acid) is a potent inhibitor of influenza virus in ferrets" Antimicrobial Agents and Chemotherapy (1995 Nov):39(11):2583-4.

Rylander R and Lin R "(1—>3)-beta-D-glucan - relationship to indoor air-related symptoms, allergy and asthma" Toxicology Nov 2000:152(1-3):47-52.

Sanchez, A et al. "Role of sugars in human neutrophilic phagocytosis" American Journal of Clinical Nutrition (1973):26:1180.

Sato, R et al. "Substances reactive with mannose-binding protein (lvIBP) in sera of patients with rheumatoid arthritis" Ind Jour Med Sci (1997):43:99-111.

See, D et al. The in vitro immunomodulatory effects of glyconutrients on peripheral blood mononuclear cells of patients with chronic fatigue syndrome" Integrative Physiological and Behavioral Science (1998 Jul-Sep):33(3):280-7.

Smith, B et al. "Analysis of inhibitor binding in influenza virus neuraminidase" Protein Science (2001 Apr):10(4):689-96.

Soltys J et al "Modulation of endotoxin- and enterotoxin-induced cytokine release by in vivo treatment with beta- (1,6)-branched beta- (1,3)-glucan" Infectious Immunology Jan1999;67(1):244-52.

Somasundaram, K and Ganguly, A "Gastric mucosal protection during restraint stress in rats: alteration in gastric adherent mucus and dissolved mucus in gastric secretion" Hepatogstroenterology (1985 Feb): 32(1):24-6.

Stuart, R et al "Upregulation of phagocytosis and candidicidal activity of macrophages exposed to the immunostimulant acemarinan" International Journal of Immunopharmacology (1997):19(2):75-82.

Sullivan, K et al. "Mannose-binding protein genetic polymorphisms in black patents with systemci lupus erythematosus" Arth and Rheumatism (Dec. 1996): 39:12, 2046-51.

Sveinbjornsson B et al "Inhibition of establishment and growth of mouse liver metastases after treatment with interferon gamma and beta-1, 3-D-glucan" Hepatology May1998:27(5):1241-8

Tate, C and Blakely, R "The effect of N-linked glycosylation on activity of the Na(+)- and Cl(-)-dependent serotonin transporter expressed using recombinant baculovirus in insect cells". J.Blol.Clzein. (1994):269(42):26303-26310.

Tazawa K, et al "Anticarcinogenic action of apple pectin on fecal enzyme activities and mucosal or portal prostaglandin E2 levels in experimental rat colon carcinogenesis" Journal of Experimental Clinical Cancer Research 1997 Mar:;16(1):33-8.

Teas J "The dietary intake of Laminarin, a brown seaweed, and breast cancer prevention" Nutrition and Cancer. 1983:4(3):217-22.

Tertov, V et al. "Carbohydrate composition of native and desialylated low density lipoproteins in the plasma of patients with coronary atherosclerosis" Kardiologiia (1992 Sep):32(9-10):57-61.

Trautwein E et al "Effect of different varieties of pectin and guar gum on plasma, hepatic and biliary lipids and cholesterol gallstone formation in hamsters fed on high-cholesterol diets" British Journal of Nutrition 1998 May;79(5):463-71.

Vlietinck, A et al. "Plant-derived leading compounds for chemotherapy of human immunodeficiency virus (HIV) infection" Planta Medica (1998 Mar):64(2):97-109.

Wakui A et al "Randomized study of lentinan on patients with advanced gastric and colorectal cancer" Tohoku Lentinan Study Group Gan To Kagaku Ryoho. Apr1986:13(4 Pt 1):1050-9.

Warczynski, P et al. "Prevention of hepatic metastases by liver lectin blocking with D-galactose in colon cancer patients. A prospectively randomized clinical trial" Anticancer Research (1997 Mar-Apr):17(2B):1223-6.

Warit, S et al. "Glycosylation deficiency phenotypes resulting from depletion of GDP-mannose pyrophosphorylase in two yeast species" Molecular Microbiology (2000 Jun):;36(5):1156-66.

Wasser S and Weis A "Therapeutic effects of substances occurring in higher Basidiomycetes mushrooms: a modern perspective" Critical Reviews of Immunology 1999:19(1):65-96.

White, M et al. "Enhanced antiviral and opsonic activity of a human mannose-binding lectin and surfactant protein D chimera" Journal of Immunology (2000 Aug 15):165(4):2108-15.

Wilke,W " Fibromyalgia. Recognizing and addressing the multiple Interrelated factors" Postgraduate Medicine (1996):100(1):153-156.

Wolff, H et al. "Adherence of Escherichia coli to sperm: a mannose mediated phenomenon leading to agglutination of sperm and E. coli" Fertility and Sterility (1993 Jul):60(1):154-8.

Yaqoob, P "Monounsaturated fats and immune function" Proc Nutr Soc (1998):57:511–20.

Yeatman, T et al "Biliary Glycoprotein Is Overexpressed in Human Colon Cancer Cells With High Metastatic Potential" Journal of Gastrointestinal Surgery (1997 May):1(3):292-298.

About the Author

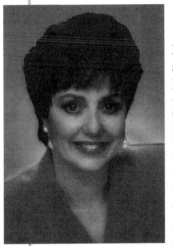

RITA ELKINS, M.H., has worked as an author and research specialist in the health field for the last ten years, and possesses a strong background in both conventional and alternative health therapies. She is the author of numerous books, including *Solving the Depression Puzzle,* which provides an in-depth look at overcoming the complex problem of depression, *The Pocket Herbal Reference, The Complete Fiber Fact Book,* and *The Herbal Emergency Guide.* Rita has also authored dozens of booklets exploring the documented value of natural supplements like SAMe, noni, blue-green algae, chitosan, stevia and many more. She received an honorary Master Herbalist Degree from the College of Holistic Health and Healing in 1994.

Rita is frequently consulted for the formulation of herbal blends and has recently joined the 4-Life Research Medical Advisory Board. She is a regular contributor to *Let's Live* and *Great Life* magazines and is a frequent host on radio talk shows exploring natural health topics. She lectures nationwide on the science behind natural compounds and collaborates with medical doctors on various projects. Rita's publications and lectures have been used by companies like Nature's Sunshine, 4-Life Research, Enrich, NuSkin, and Nutraceutical to support the credibility of natural and integrative health therapies. She recently co-authored *Soy Smart Health* with *New York Times'* best-selling author Neil Solomon, M.D.

Rita resides in Utah, is married, and has two daughters and two granddaughters.

Woodland Health Series

*Definitive Natural Health Information
At Your Fingertips!*

The Woodland Health Series offers a comprehensive array of single topic booklets, covering subjects from fibromyalgia to green tea to acupressure. If you enjoyed this title, look for other WHS titles at your local health-food store, or contact us. Complete and mail (or fax) us the coupon below and receive the complete Woodland catalog and order form—free!

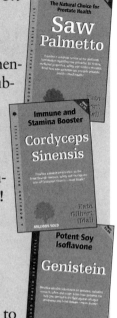

Or . . .

- Call us toll-free at **(800) 777-2665**
- Visit our website
  (www.woodlandpublishing.com)
- Fax the coupon (and other correspondence) to
  (801) 785-8511
